The Extra Button

Background

In 2008 my husband and I were faced with the choice of whether to forgo having children or opt for donor conception. It was a privilege to have such a choice. At the time it was a difficult decision for us, but if you are reading this book, it may be a choice you are familiar with.

Even before our twins were born, we faced another decision – when, how and indeed, if we tell our children. My husband and I both agreed that we would start discussing donor conception with them from an early age so that it might avoid an unnecessary shock later in life.

It's not an easy concept to grasp as a child. More difficult to understand in many ways than adoption or some other forms of assisted conception. As a trained teacher, I knew that storytelling would be one of the most powerful ways to explain a tricky topic such as this and I promised my unborn twins that I would write a book for them, introducing them to the concept of donor conception from a very early age.

I have tried to use storytelling to provide a metaphor for the facts of donor conception so that children can start to understand what it means. I also hope this story provides reassurance to donor conception children that they are loved very much by their parent (s), regardless of their genetic connection. Because being a parent is a great deal more than providing the genes. It's also about being there, side-by-side with the child(ren) as they grow up, loving them and nurturing them to adulthood and beyond.

Our story can be found on www.donorconception.com.au

To Jasper & Charlotte

Illustrations by Fefe

Somewhere in the gingerbread
village lived two gingerbreads
called Benny and Rose.

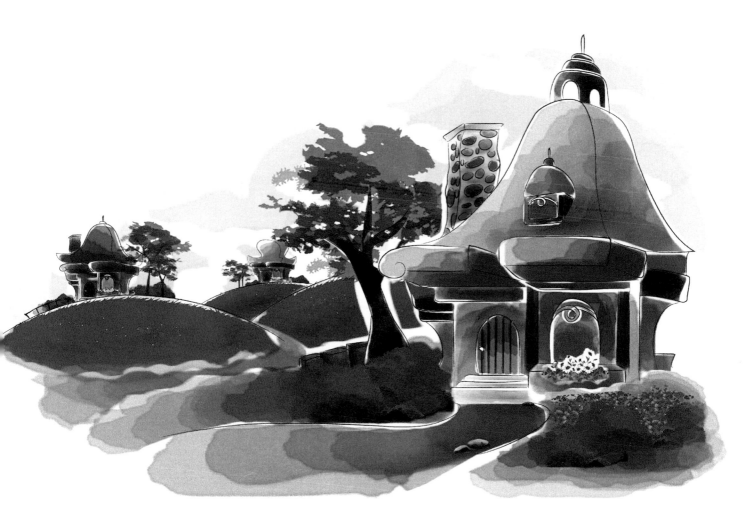

Benny and Rose had lots of friends and they had a happy life. But what they wanted more than anything was to have children of their own.

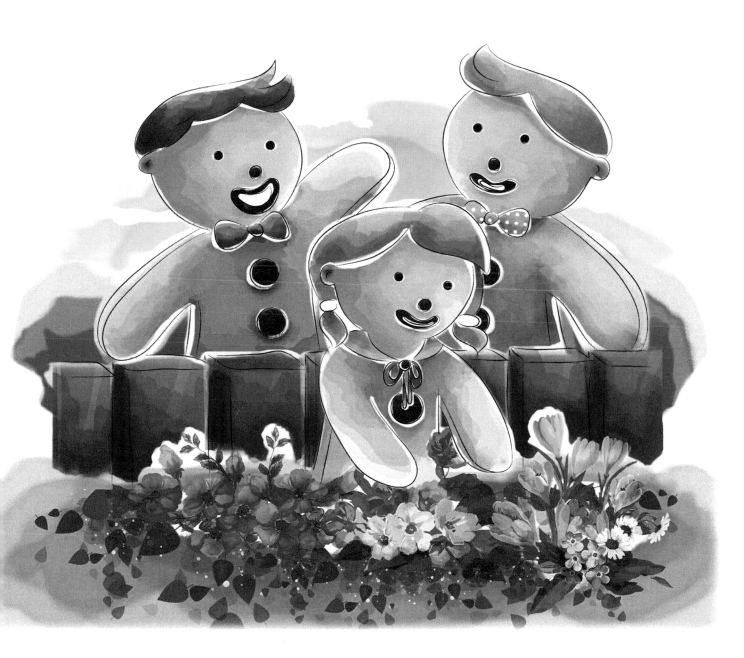

When a mummy and a daddy gingerbread wanted to have a baby, they each had to give one button to make the baby. But Rose only had one button. She didn't have an extra one to give.

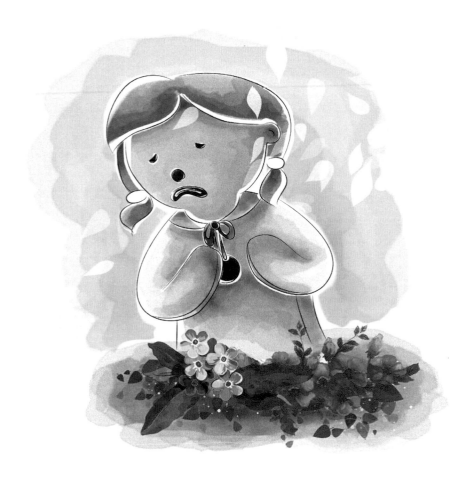

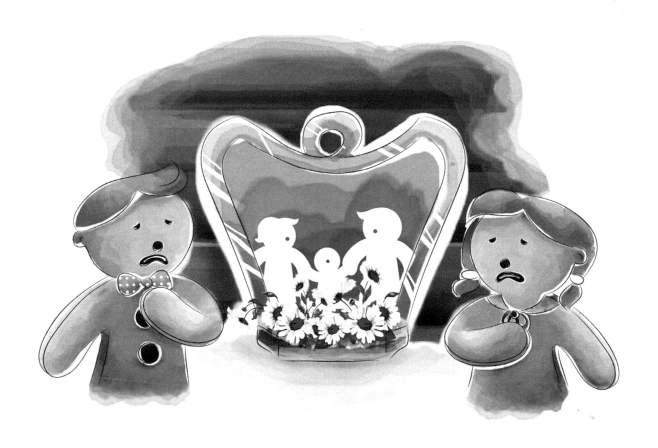

$\mathfrak{M}$ost evenings, they would eat dinner

then walk through the village. As Rose

passed by houses of families with children,

the sounds of their laughter and singing

would bring tears to her eyes.

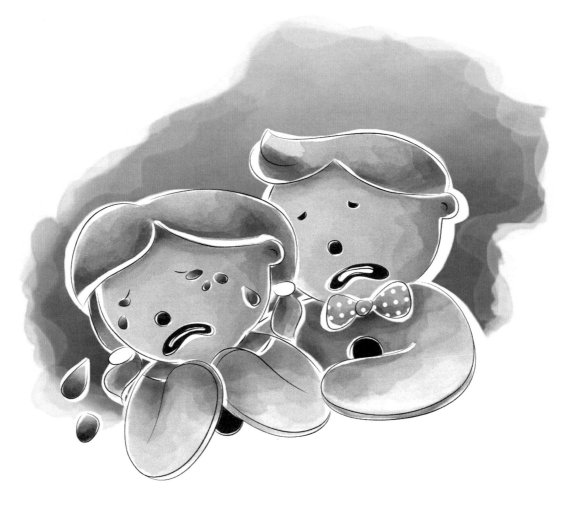

"Oh Benny, I want to have children so badly," she would say. Benny would only nod. He had the same wish. But what could they do? They didn't have enough buttons to make a baby.

Rose's friend, Heather, knew they were unhappy. She suggested they talk to the village wise man about their wish. They were willing to try anything so they agreed.

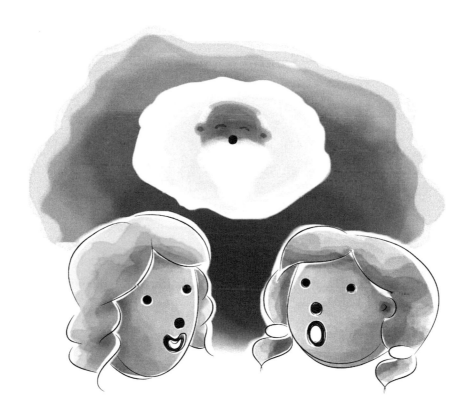

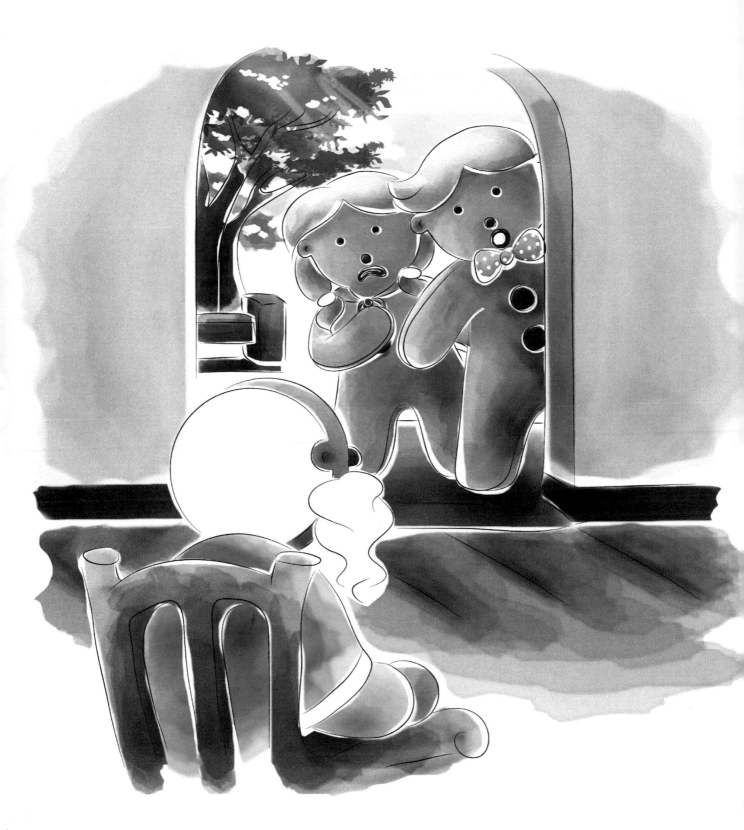

They went to the wise man's little house and found him sitting in an old wooden chair. He peered at them and listened while they told him how they really wanted to have a child.

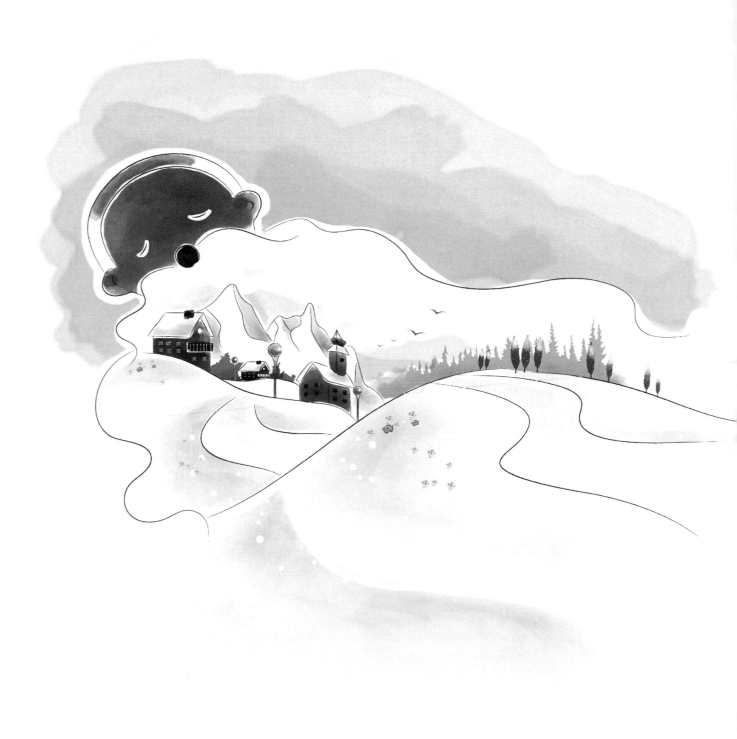

When they finished, the old man coughed loudly and then started speaking in a croaky old voice.

"Long ago, there was a story about a village near the top of Brown Mountain," he told them.

"It was said that some of the women there have three buttons. Perhaps that's where you can find your answer." Then he fell asleep.

Brown Mountain was so far away, but Rose and Benny were ready to do anything to make their baby. They filled up their packs and headed out towards the great mountain which loomed in the distance. It looked like it was too far away to ever get there, but they were determined to try.

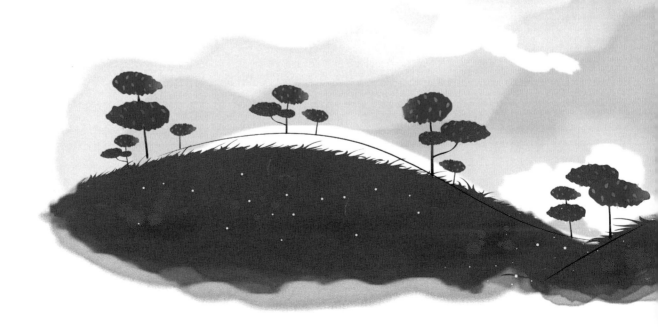

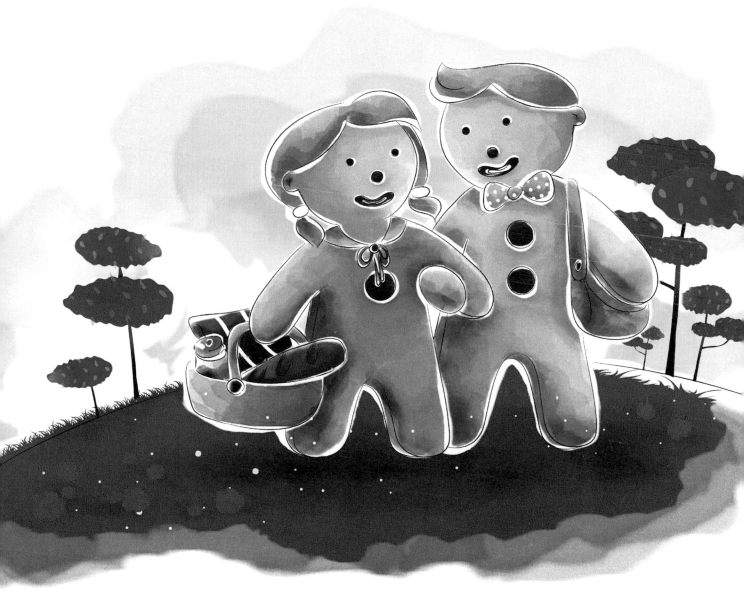

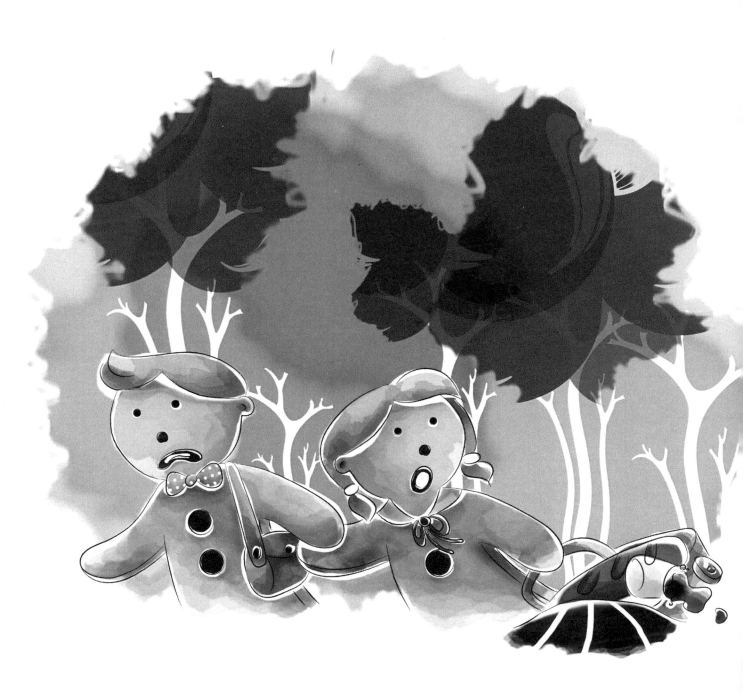

They walked for days over the grassy hills. One day they came to the edge of a deep forest.

"It's pretty dark in there, Benny," said Rose.

"It sure is, but we'll find our way," said Benny.

After they had passed through the forest they began to hear a rumbling sound in the distance. They walked on and the sound got louder. "It's a river!" said Rose.

They came to a steep gorge and peered over the edge. White-water roared below them.

"I wouldn't want to get dunked in there! I can't swim," exclaimed Benny.

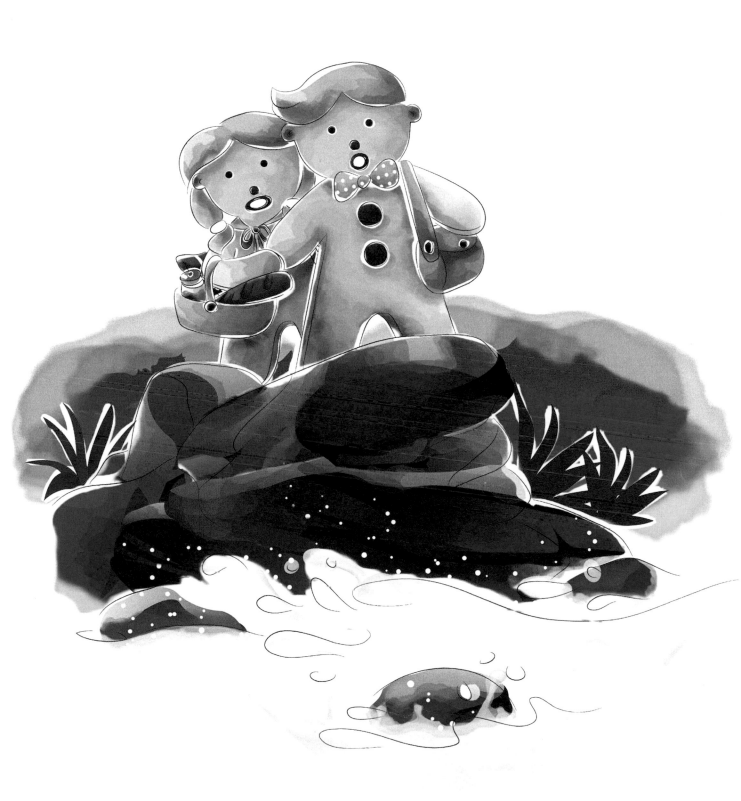

Near them was a rickety old wooden bridge. "I don't think we can walk across that," said Benny. "We have to cross if we want to get that button," said Rose. "Come on!" She took Benny's hand and carefully stepped onto the bridge.

They walked slowly, with the bridge creaking and swaying over the rushing water, but together they got to the other side.

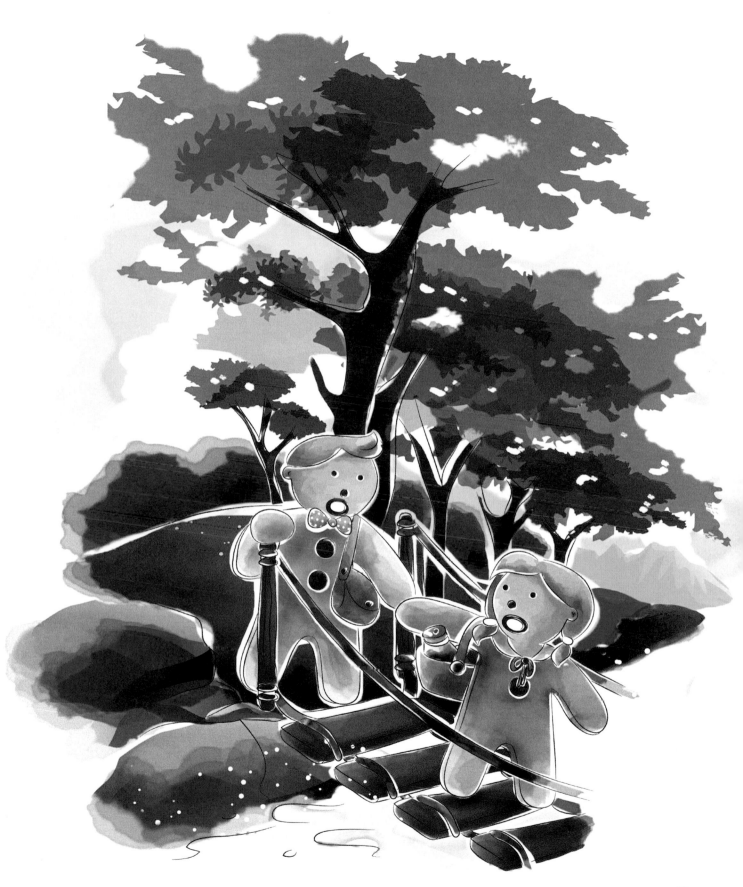

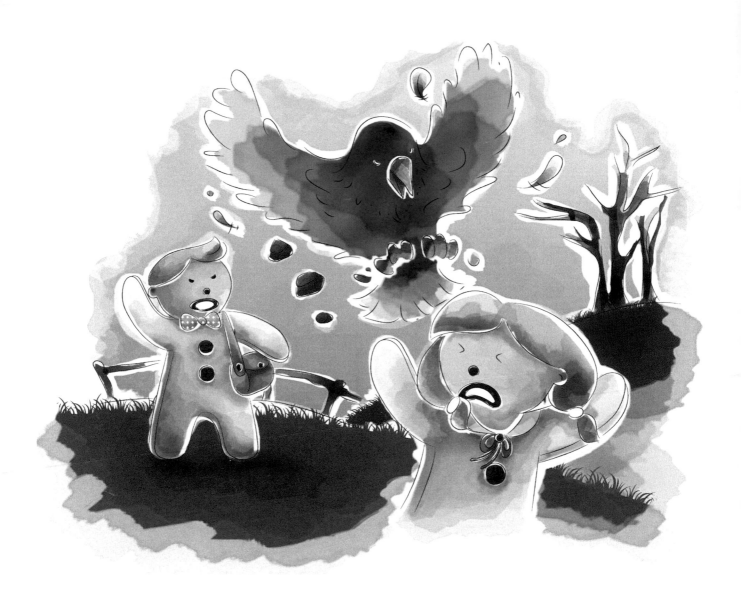

"That was scary, but we made it," said Benny.

"Wait, what's that sound?" asked Rose.

"It's a bird. Run!"

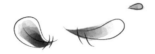

A big black bird swooped down from the sky heading straight towards them. Benny quickly picked up some brown rocks and threw them at the bird until it finally flew away and Rose was safe again.

Brown rocks - they had finally reached Brown Mountain! The mountain was steep and soon they were climbing over boulders and up steep slopes.

When they felt too tired to carry on, they smiled at each other and whistled happy tunes to keep themselves going. "I hope there's really an extra button for us up there," said Rose.

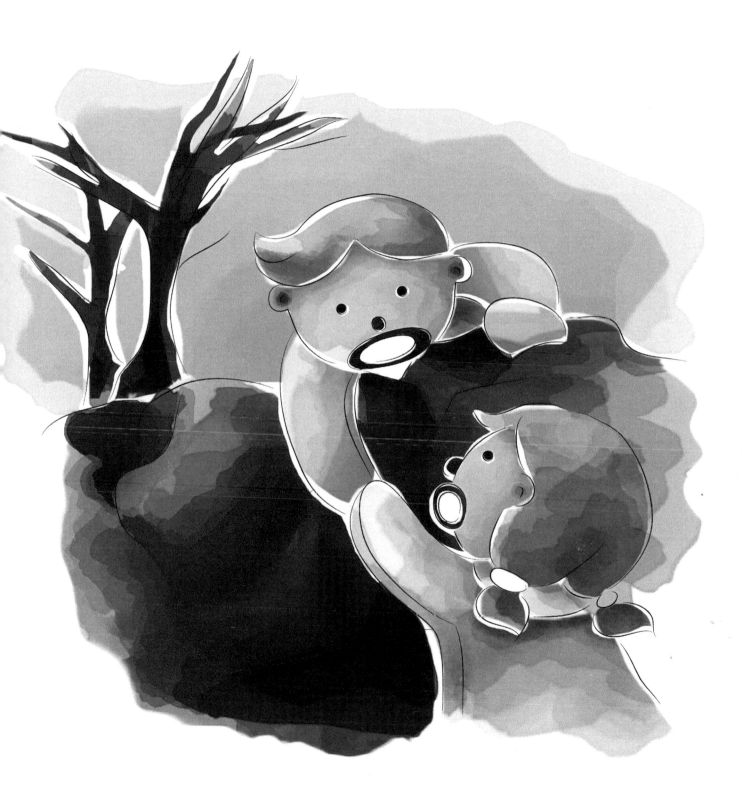

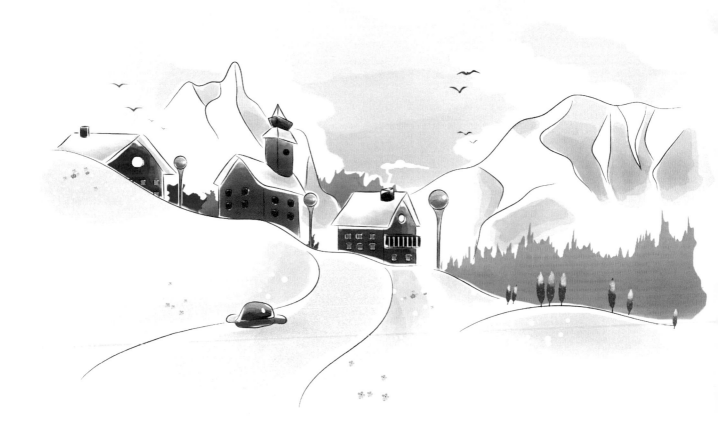

At the top of the mountain they saw
what they had come searching for.
They hiked into a small village full of
strange-looking houses.

$\mathfrak{M}$any people came outside to look at them. Rose found her courage and spoke,

"We've come a long way to find a button to help us make our baby. Can you help us?"

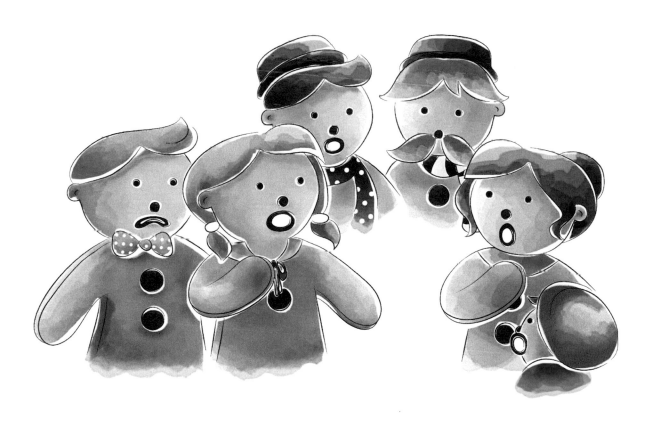

One man smiled and took Rose's hand. "Don't worry, I think I have an answer to your problem."

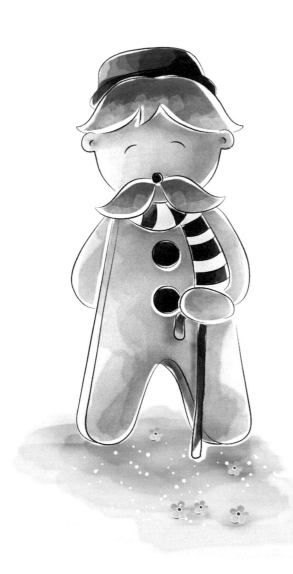

He led them to a big house and there standing in front of it was a woman with three buttons!

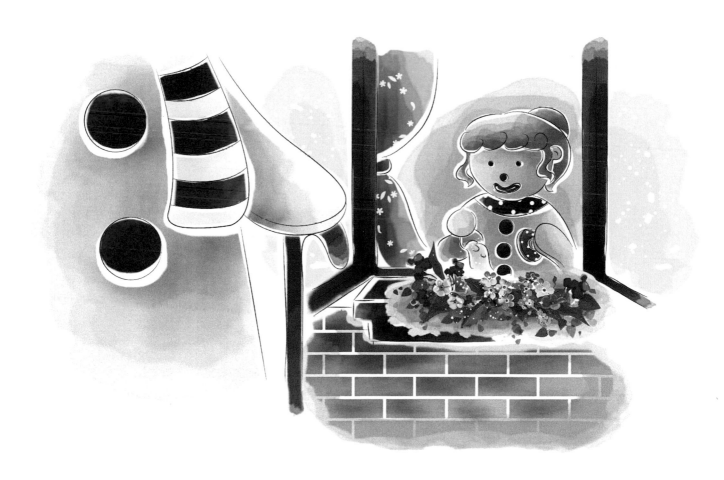

Benny and Rose told her their story. When they finished, she smiled a great big smile and said,

"You have so much strength and love to give to a child. I want you to have my extra button. Please take it."

Rose was so happy she could burst! She gave the woman a big hug and the woman gave her a beautiful red button, placing it onto Rose's tummy to grow safely. She and Benny could finally make their dream come true.

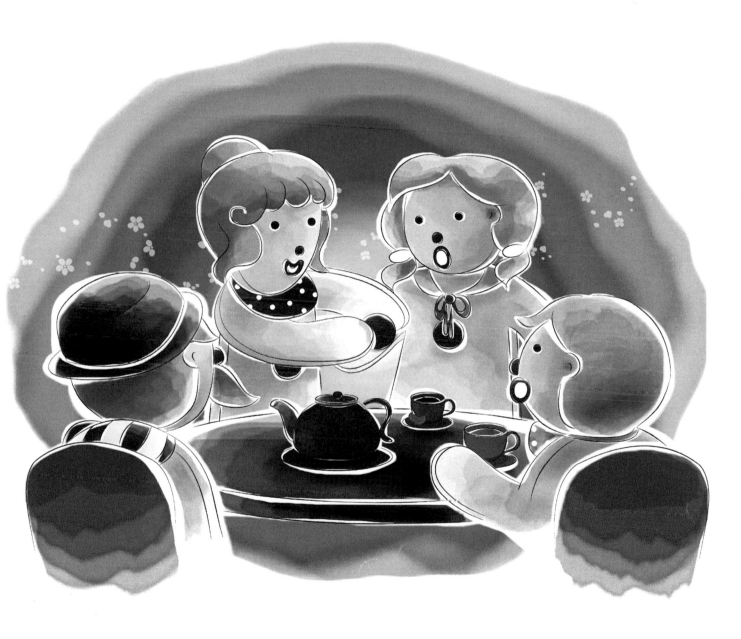

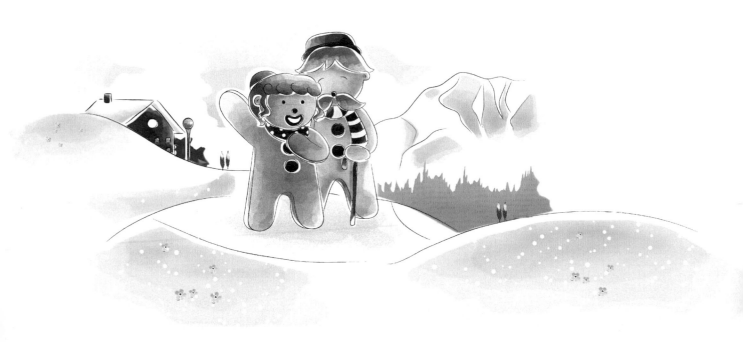

They said goodbye to the kind people on the mountain and set off for home.

They walked for days and days, but that didn't bother them at all. They thought only about keeping their unborn baby safe and about how happy they would be once it was born. They whistled and hummed happy songs the whole way home.

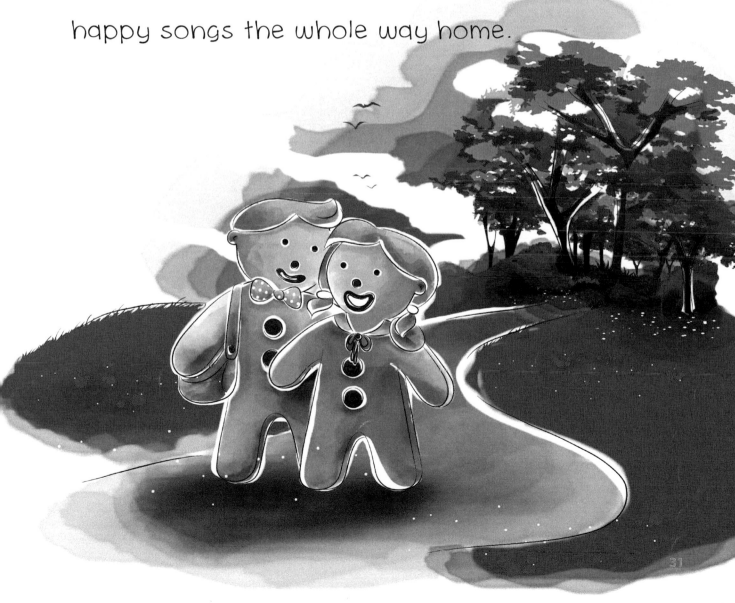

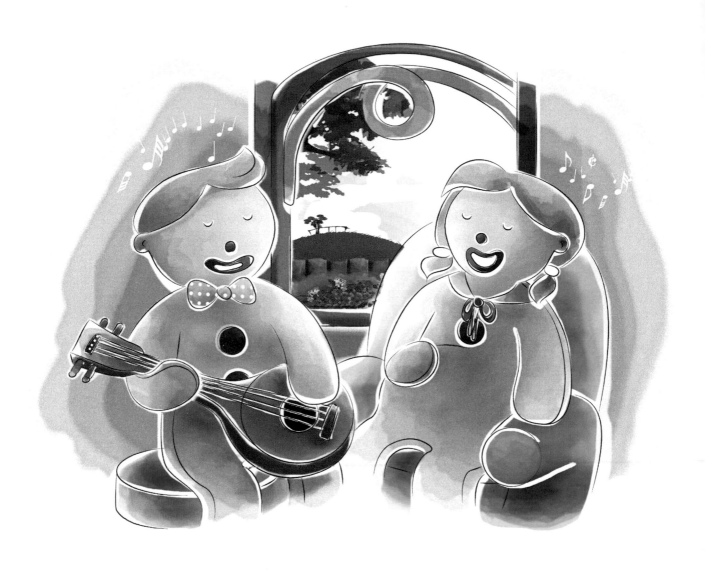

When Rose and Benny arrived home, the whole village greeted them. Everyone could see from their faces that they had found the button they had been hoping for.

Benny learned to play the guitar and every day he and Rose would sing to the baby in Rose's tummy. After a few months, Rose gave birth to a beautiful little boy and they named him Bertie.

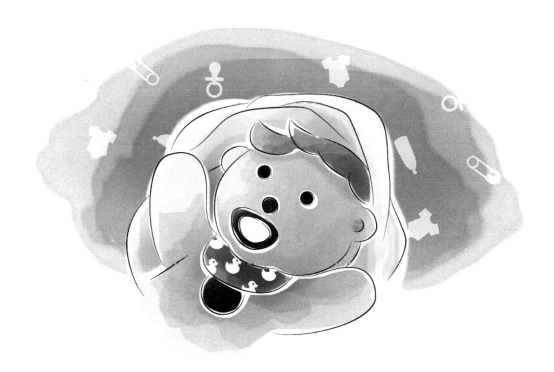

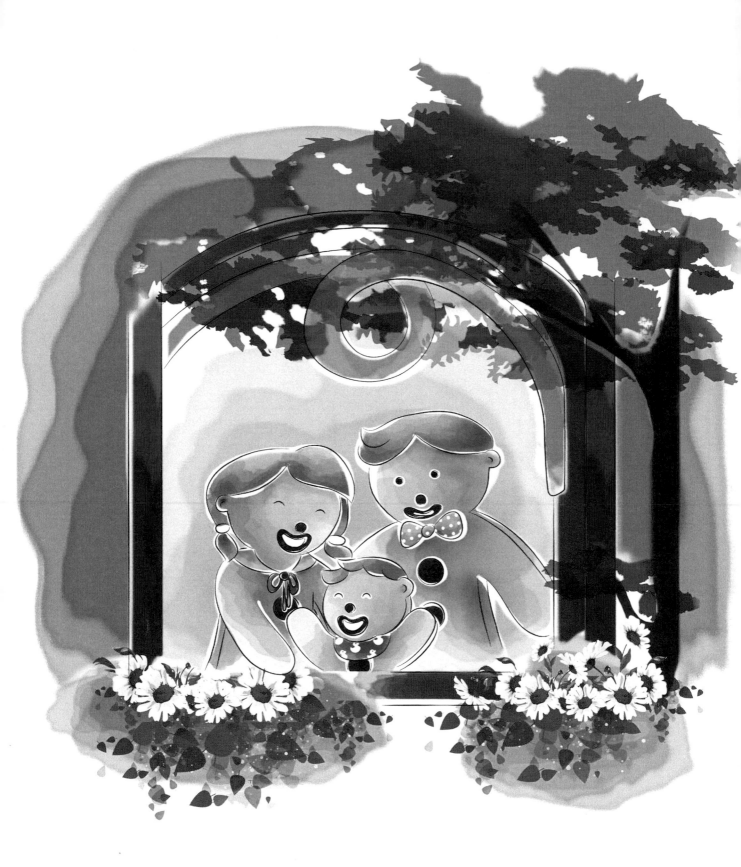

As Bertie grew up, Benny and Rose loved him more than anything, and then some.

After their journey, Benny and Rose no longer like to walk much anymore, but if you happen to be in their village and walk by their house in the evening, you'll hear the sounds of music and laughter floating through the air - the sounds of the happiest family on earth.

The end

National Library of Australia Cataloguing-in-Publication entry (paperback):

Author:	Blundell, Jules, author.
Title:	The extra button / Jules Blundell ; Fefe, illustrator.
ISBN:	9780992418205 (paperback)
Target Audience:	For primary school age.
Subjects:	Parents – Juvenile fiction.
	Childbirth – Juvenile fiction.
Other Authors/ Contributors:	Fefe, illustrator.
Dewey Number:	A823.4

Printed in Australia by Lightning Source
Typeset by Michael Hanrahan Publishing Services
Illustrated by Fefe

CPSIA information can be obtained
at www.ICGtesting.com
Printed in the USA
LVXC01n1709201117
557023LV00013B/251